Chosen

What to Expect When You've Been Diagnosed with Cancer.

Michelle Tucker

Printed by KDP/Amazon.com, Inc., in the United States of America.

ISBN: 9781099067471

First printing, 2019.

KDP Self-Publishing

Contact author: mlstucker@yahoo.com

Acknowledgements

First, to Almighty God for choosing me and giving me
endurance and strength to push the envelope on so many levels,
and for making me trust my intuition and believe in myself!
Secondly, this book is dedicated to my three amazing children,
Adam, Sarah, and Trinity. You've all made me stronger, wiser, and
taught me the meaning of unconditional love. I love you to the
moon and back!

To my mom, brother, and sister Thank you for standing beside
me on my walk of life and always picking up the phone when I call
to ramble. To my father in heaven, thank you for helping shape
me into the woman I've become. To my grandma Phyllis, who is
also watching from the skies above, thank you for your love,
encouragement, and guidance, as I know that I talked your head off
with countless phone calls before your left our earth.

To my editor and friend, you know who you are, thank you for
believing in me. My warmest "thank you" from the bottom of my
heart.

And finally, to my belated husband, Allen. Thank you for loving me, never judging me, and for just being you. Until we meet again.

Chosen

CONTENTS
TABLE OF CONTENTS

1 A Little about Me   1

2 Are You Kidding Me?   10

3 The Oncologist   21

4 Sugar, EMF's Radiation, and Chemotherapy   29

5 Questions and Answers   35

6 Doctor Lingo   43

7 The First Oncologist Appointment   56

8 Michelle's Tips to Help Get you Through the Day   61

One

A Little About Me

My name is Michelle. I am a Registered Nurse with a vast amount of medical experience under my belt. I didn't begin as a nurse, but first began my career in physical therapy. I wanted to blossom out so I felt nursing was a career which I feel called to do as touching the lives of others and making a positive impact is extremely rewarding. My heart is overjoyed when I make just one person's day a little brighter. I'm a tattoo artist who believes in giving back to my fellow sisters and brothers who undergo mastectomies by tattooing back the areolas, making the survivors feel beautiful and whole again. I call this the ICING ON THE CAKE! I believe we are all here for a purpose on God's beautiful Earth, and with that in mind, we all have a function, a reason, and an incredible life that we are given to live. Our lives are full of up's and down's, twists and turns, some faster than others, and some seem like they are on a slow path. But whatever maybe we are ALL here on this beautiful journey called Life!

1

A glimpse of my life just for insight...

I am the mother of three amazing children, one boy and two daughters and our family German shepherd. I am a three-time survivor of breast cancer, thyroid cancer, and I am currently going thru pancreatic cancer treatment. I can honestly tell you I love my children with my entire heart and soul. I am a widow to the most loving husband, in my eye's, that God ever created. And, yep, you guessed it, he lost his battle with cancer in just under seven weeks from diagnosis.

After the passing of my husband our lives had been changed forever; we were not prepared for this at all. But who is RIGHT? We had literally just canceled his life insurance plan and was advised to re-up a new-improved version December 1, 2009. You're probably wondering why? Well, here it is per the advice of our insurance agent, let's call him, Rick, for the purpose of my story. Rick stated to cancel and re-up would be a huge benefit for us because we could raise the amount, we currently had in place in the event of something like this happening. He proceeded to sell us on the purposed offer from 50k to 250k! Oh my, that's a huge difference in payouts if you really think about it for a minute. Rick rattled on saying this reasoning would be a huge benefit for our family. Truth be told, my husband was a little on the heavy side. I mean let's face it, without working out like crazy and watching every bite we put in our mouths, most of us are not at our high school skinny weight. With that in mind my husband had set a goal and he achieved it. He lost 50 pounds and if he proved to hold the weight off for one year, which he did, we could raise the life insurance amounts. I mean who in their right mind wouldn't do that! So, under the direction of Rick, we went ahead and canceled our current plan on November 1, 2009. Rick, our charming insurance agent assured us that 30 days later we would be on a new and improved policy. Here's the kicker—are you ready? Just eleven days later yep eleven short days later Allen wasn't feeling well. I recognized this wasn't typical flu-like symptoms. This was different, and my radar was up per my intuition. I had just walked in the door from working the night shift at Gilbert Hospital. I sent my husband to the hospital to get checked in while I took a quick shower.

Allen underwent an MRI on November 11, 2009. That test prompted a call to a general surgeon who stated his case, from what he could tell on the films, looked to be relatively simple they would just surgically remove his stomach and create a passage and a new way to process his food intake system. He sent us over to the radiology department and Allen underwent a paracentesis and biopsy to give the surgeon a quick look at any other difficulties that may not have shown on his scan. With the physician's reassurance, we were told to go home and await his call. So, as obedient patients that we were, we headed home to try and have a normal dinner time with my children. Within three hours from our return home, my phone rang, and my heart sunk to the bottom of my stomach. Each call was from the surgeon. Each call started with, "Michelle, we have a preliminary diagnosis for your husband." Within fifteen minutes the diagnosis became evident that my strong, amazing, unstoppable, husband was going in for a huge battle of his lifetime. I immediately called his mom, who lived out of state and gave her the information I had on hand. With much persuasion, she agreed to come out for his surgery. I just knew in my gut, this wasn't going to go as smoothly as they were portraying it to be. Boy, I was right! Twenty-two minutes into surgery, the main surgeon came out of the operating room and asked to speak quietly to me. I felt like my heart had stopped! He gave me the news that, blah, blah, blah, you know, the "I'm sorry speech", but truly he stated he had surgically opened my husband's abdomen and the cancer was so great that there was nothing they could do but close him back up with stitches and staples. My mind was racing in so many directions. After awakening from the recovery room, we soon meant an oncologist that insisted she could help. So, Allen being the wonderful man he is, decided to take her advice and receive chemotherapy treatments. But I stood my ground, questioning the hell out of her and raising as much cain as I could with the back-to-back treatments. Allen thought she was giving him a chance and agreed to go forward. So, the first treatment was on December 23rd and the next on December 24th.

After the second chemotherapy treatment, I was able to take

him home to try and have some kind of Christmas holiday with our kids. Allen was a champ on Christmas morning. He pushed through his shakiness and came out to the couch to watch our children open their Christmas gifts that were, unbeknownst to me, mostly from volunteers that my dear friend, Patty, had arranged. We made it through the day, and with a few visits back and forth to the hospital, one of those times, was when my brother-in-law, helped get Allen in the truck and then raced down the freeway driving what seemed to be 100 miles per hour, to rule out a blood clot in Allen's leg.

Allen remained strong as a bull until the night of January 4th. I had showered him and got him sitting in a chair next to our bed. I took four steps out of our bedroom and then I had the strongest, weird feeling to turn back to check on him. He had a look of terror on his face. We rushed him to the hospital where he was immediately admitted into the ICU. I knew this wasn't good. Allen was able to talk to me and stated he was scared and to always remember our wedding day as it was the happiest day of his life. Can you imagine how that felt? I felt like I had been kicked in the gut because I knew now, he knew.

I requested a pastor to come and pray over him for a peaceful transition. My father, mother-in-law, and I were all in his room for his final hours. Allen's physician that was on call, Dr. P., was amazing during this most difficult time. Allen didn't want to leave this earth yet, he had a lot to do still, but our almighty God needed him, so he called him home, January 5th, 2010. The days after seemed like such a blur, I honestly remember things in a foggy way.

A check from Allen's life insurance plan from his current employer was sent and then pulled back due to an administration error. Their Human Resource department had gone through some changes a few months prior and the employees had to sign new forms. So, being the obedient employee that he was, he did sign but forgot to date them! Can you believe that! How did human resources not catch that silly mistake! Did they not have their eyes working properly that day, and where did their checks and balances accountability come into play! Needless to say, I had to send the check back. So here I am, recent widow head spinning, feeling like I was in fog and couldn't even fathom what was happening. Being a young, inexperienced wife, I did what they said, and sent the check back letting them know that mistakes like this should never, ever, happen. Heck, we were a young family raising our children, this wasn't going to happen to us.

We were living life to the fullest and had just got back from an incredible weekend in San Diego celebrating my son's 13th birthday together making memories. My husband made a last-minute decision, which I was shocked because I was the planner in our family for excursions not him. He had the trip all planned in his amazing head exactly what we were going to go do.

You see I worked nights at the local hospital as a charge nurse. I had just come home from my night shift and he was standing in the doorway with the biggest smile ever with the kids and suitcases packed and said, "Hi! How was your night?" Before I could answer his question, he said: "Let's go have some fun!" That weekend will forever be ingrained into my memory bank. We laughed so hard our stomachs hurt, we played with the kids, went to SeaWorld, and just had an over-all blast together.

He spent money like it was no object, which I have to share with you; this was really out of the norm. That should've been my clue, looking back makes you wonder if deep down inside he knew something wasn't right. Nah, he had just had a physical and passed with flying colors and I was with him on his appointment. Allen was a saver when it came to money matters. After our return home in the blink of an eye, our lives changed forever. I would find myself dazed and actually pinch myself to see if what was happening was a dream or was, I really living through this roller coaster ride we commonly refer to as life. We were forced to learn how to be a family unit with just the four of us and our beloved Lab, Jasmine. The reality of hearing that you are going to go into the battle of your life and FIGHT to WIN this against this ugly Beast is one that none of us humans should ever have to endure.

Two

Are you kidding me?!

Just as we're plugging along in this new way of life, I treated myself and purchased a few new bras. As most of us ladies do, I washed them and placed in the dresser drawer until a later date.

You're probably wondering why do we need to know this? Hold on, here we go! It was three days later that my daughter wasn't feeling well. I got a call from the school assistant that my daughter complained about her tummy ache, and she had a fever and a cough that progressed to sounding like a seal-like bark. Now I will admit being a nurse I am not, I repeat I am not, the mom that runs to the doctor's office for every little sniffle. Heck, I respond to my kids on a regular basis by asking, "Is it broke? Bleeding? Hurt as you've never experienced before?" If they answer, no to all these questions, then I tell them to dust yourself off and let's go! I know that sounds harsh to some but I just need them to be strong and brush off the little scrapes and get back up! But, her seal-like barking and constant coughing continued to get worse.

I decided to take her into our local primary care physician's office. It here is where it starts. The doctor examined my daughter, prescribed antibiotics, cough syrup, so she could get some relief and sleep at night, along with a steroid, and an inhaler to be on the safe side. She stated my daughter had caught the bug and it is a bad one. I began to gear up for unplanned but necessary downtime including going over the recipe for my homemade chicken noodle soup, good movies, and if she was awake, lots of cuddling time with mom. But it doesn't end there dear reader. Can you believe the PCP, being the observant person, she was, noticed I had readjusted my bra on the left side several times?

Cleverly, she sent my daughter down the hall to pick out her stickers for good behavior, and then turned to me to ask me why I was fidgeting with my bra. I proceeded to give her some song and dance that it was just the new bra's cleavage-making wires that were poking me. Without much delay, I found myself on the examining table. I decided to appease her and get it over with as quick as possible. I mean seriously, it was nothing!

As I stared off into space, she knew I was nervous and asked me to quiet my mind for a minute. Without further ado, she asked if she could look at the left side where the wire was bothering me. She began her examination and then gave me that LOOK! You know that look of, oh dear—I'm sorry! I know you all know what I'm referring to—something like the look your mother would give you and you knew you were busted.

I smiled trying to keep positive, I asked her "What's up? Do I need to toss out this brand-new cleavage-booming bra already? "I wasn't getting off that easy. She quickly handed me a request to go have a mammogram and then I explained to her I had already undergone a partial mastectomy and radiation treatments back in 2007-2008 for breast cancer. I think she literally could see the wheels in my head spinning. She made a call to the imaging center and changed the order to a STAT MRI of the breast. My daughter returned so our conversation stopped and I refocused on her.

After leaving the office, I immediately called the Imaging center to confirm and give insurance information. They made my appointment for 5:45 P.M., that same night. I got my daughter home and started her medications and away I went to get my MRI.

The next morning, my phone rang and low and behold it was the primary care's office. It was only 7:15 in the morning, why would my doctor be calling so early? Did they even have their computer son or have their first cup of coffee?

After identifying herself on the phone, she said, "My dear, I believe you are going to endure another mountain to climb. This one will be tough, but stay focused and you can do it." WHAT? Are you kidding me? Are you sure you have the right woman? After what seemed to be a five-minute pause in our conversation, she gave me a few names and numbers of recommended Oncologists close to where I lived. Well, if I didn't understand her sentence structure message before, I can surely tell you the word O-N-C-O-L-O-G-I-S-T gives you a crystal-clear picture that something is about to go down!

I got off the phone and honestly, I don't even recall ending the call. This was Thanksgiving weekend and we were already not too fond of this holiday because the previous Thanksgiving my husband was in the hospital and on the Thanksgiving Day the physician requested me to have my sister bring in our kids to say goodbye to their father as he didn't think he would make it to Christ.

Immediately after that call, I was in a very stunned state of mind. I remember walking out to my front porch with tears streaming down my face. I found myself yelling to the bluest sky ever, Wow! Haven't we had enough? Why us again? You could've picked diagonally someone else. I shed a few more tears and then put on my "poker" face and went back inside. I had to remember that I had made a promise to myself after my recent changes in my life that my demeanor was to maintain a calm home environment for my children at all costs.

Moving forward and thinking of my family first, I wrestled with the thought of how was I going to keep it together and not burst into tears until I am able to see the oncologist and hear what he/she has to say? It was that moment I decided I would keep my worries, thoughts, and questions, that were running around wildly in my head to myself. I bargained with myself to keep quiet until I had more concrete evidence and a plan of action and attack outlined. You see, I would have loved to go cry on my mom's shoulders, or dad, sister, or my brother, but in the strangest way, I felt guilty for just leaning on everyone just 10 months ago during the passing of my beloved husband.

A few days later I was able to get into the Oncologist office; the news was a little worse than I imagined. I, Michelle a brand-new widow and mom of three, received the news that I had a stage 2spot on the left breast and a stage 3 spot on the right breast. Which equals re-current breast cancer. I recall staring with a blank expression on my face while the oncologist spoke.

My heart pounded and my stomach was turning upside down. It's a miracle I didn't toss my cookies in his office at the very moment. I instantly had the most nauseous feeling overwhelm me. As he continued to talk, it felt like I was in a tunnel as his words sounded muffled. He would stop talking and just look at me. In my mind, I would continue to just stare at him. And then it was on—I began firing questions off to him: How could this be? Why is this happening? I believed I was a compliant patient. Heck, I followed all the rules as far as medication and dietary changes were concerned. I even gave up Starbucks! Is this for real or is someone playing a twisted joke on me?

I had been put on the drug called, Tamoxifen. I had faithfully taken it for three plus years after my last battle with the beast. I was told that I just had to get to the five-year mark and I would be in complete remission. It was a marathon that I had been running and I was more than halfway to the finish line. I could see the light at the end of the tunnel that I had visualized over and over in my head of me running with the torch of life and breaking through the PINK ribbon at the finish line and feeling how awesome to be at five years remission and be done! Done with swallowing that pill every day and wondering what it was doing for and to me.

I envisioned people cheering, music and balloons everywhere. What a victorious day that would be in my life! At this initial appointment we discussed my treatment plan and decided on future testing and a surgical date to "look around". We came up with the initial look around date to be December 31,2010. This got me through the Christmas holiday. I didn't want this heavy burden on anyone's holiday. My mom had a very important state test she needed to take. Also, for my children, this was the first Christmas after my husband's passing and I felt like it was my job to make sure that I taught my children we were all going to be okay.

My out-of-town family was scheduled to leave first thing the same morning that I had my discovery procedure. My girlfriend, Sandy, had picked me up early and we said we had a meeting at work so there wouldn't be any questions that I'd be forced to answer. Questions of the unknown tend to get me nervous. Being in the medical field my entire life, I like to know how things work and no concrete answers didn't sit well with me or my brain.

Without missing a beat, Sandy picked me up and away we went to the hospital. During the ride we did discussed things regarding our work life, joked around about silly girl things, and before we knew it, we had arrived at the hospital in Scottsdale where Sandy patiently waited several hours for me. After recovery, I was extremely sore. Sandy carefully drove watching every little bump, and I was very grateful for her consideration.

To be completely honest with you I wasn't surprised when the results came less than 24 hours later. I admit I began to hate my phone and the numbers that were calling it. Without further fuss, I was immediately pulled back into the Chemotherapy arena once again. The chemotherapy room reminds me of a herd of cattle as all we do is sit in a large room with recliner chairs and stare at each other, the television, or we are all on our cellular devices. Honestly, in the chemotherapy infusion rooms, I actually had the blessings of meeting some really fascinating people. Heck, I even crocheted a blanket and had the pleasure of teaching a gentleman, that wanted to give his wife of 57 years something special, to personally crochet something for her birthday.

Under my doctor's recommendation, I underwent a total of seven surgeries over the next year and a half. Including a bilateral mastectomy with reconstruction. Due to scaring on the right side that caused my arm to not have the mobility to move up and down, I had to endure that procedure again. An entire hysterectomy due to being estrogen receptor +, a total thyroidectomy, and the remaining unforeseen surgeries all breast related. My gosh, if you think about it, more strangers have seen me in a vulnerable state in the surgical suite than I could count on both of my hands.

With all this in mind, I found that as cliché as it sounds, our minds control everything about us. If we hear such news and give in to the Beast, we are giving it power! Power to take over our lives. Whether we like it or not, fear and uncertainty begin to consume our every thought. For me this was not an option, no way in hell was I going to give this disease any power. Instead, I gave an eviction notice to get the hell out of my body. I was determined to win and I would not be defeated!

I will share with you this is something that some of us don't want to talk about our treatment or the disease—not because we are hiding things or keeping facts from our loved ones, I can assure you that's not it at all. It is merely the fact that we are dealing with the diagnosis as best as we can. For some, not talking about it may make it easier to endure, but for me, well, I just wanted to be thankful for the immediate minute that I was blessed to live. Discussing my illness day in and day out, I believed, was giving my malady some kind of authority and giving it power. This drained all the positive energy I had stored up in my reserve tank.

I was not going to fuel its power in any way. Like I said—I gave it notice of eviction. I felt I needed to conserve all the positive energy to fight back. Some women, continue to live our lives, putting on our make-up. We believe this makes us look and feel better when we look in the mirror, and we put on our happy face so others think that we looked good for the day. Little do they know of the emotional turbulence we are handling on the inside during this fierce life and death battle. As for me, I chose to keep my emotional pain to myself. When needed, I would give myself permission, (at short intervals), to cry in the shower. I only wanted my children to see their strong-ass resilient mother.

Three

The Oncologist

As promised, I'm sharing a few things with you that I wish, at the beginning of my treatment, the Oncologists would have divulged and openly shared. Like honestly these side effects are no secret. Are they afraid if they told us what really to expect that we would run, not walk out of their offices never to return?

But, hey, if they haven't walked in our shoes how would they know?! In my experience, physicians, for the most part, deal with what's written on paper or in a medical book. What if they just thought outside those controlled boxes?

What if they pushed back the pharmaceutical companies, and the poly-tricks involved in our healthcare system? Would more of our lives be spared? I am living proof that being your own voice and not being afraid to upset the doctor who sits at a fancy desk giving you such news. Remember how you felt when they told you x, y, or z? So where's the harm in upsetting them a little. First things first—this information is only meant to inform, empower, educate, and possibly ignite the burning urge to fill you with a bit of knowledge and understanding. It is not meant to replace your Oncologist's advice regarding your medical treatments. This will simply give you something else to think about.

The Power of Your Mind...

What cancer is: a journey and a battle.

What cancer is NOT: a life sentence.

A wise man once told me, "Your mind is a very powerful tool. "There is no stronger statement. Allow me to empower you with knowledge and give you the will to fight! Let me ease your mind and realize cancer is not your fault. Stand up and make a difference because you are stronger than you think!

At Beijing medical university, the students were told, "One-third of patients die of the psychological shock of being told by a doctor that they have cancer. Another third died from the negative effects of chemotherapy and radiation. The last third simply die.

"Why is that? Your mind can determine your outcome. Think positive and you will receive positive outcomes. Remember when you went on that job interview you really wanted? You thought long and hard, sending out positive vibes to the universe, and low and behold, you actually got the call!

Cancer is Big Business

The politics of chemotherapy are REAL. There are pharmaceutical companies involved, patents on medications, scientists, testing in labs, Oncologists, FDA, drug reps, and the list goes on. Did you ever wonder or ponder about the treatment protocol regimen your doctor prescribed had the potential to actually increase the likelihood that in the future you would become a repeat customer to the Oncology office? Studies have proven this to be true. That's job security in my book!

Little Known Facts You Should Be Aware Of:

At the beginning of the last century, one person in twenty would get cancer. In the 1940's it was one out of every sixteen. In 1970, it was one out of every ten. Today, the World Health

Organization just released its estimate that 18.1 million new cancer cases will be diagnosed around the world. This is up from the 14.1 million new cases and 8.2 million deaths reported back in 2012. Today, one out of three people will be diagnosed in their life span. I pose the question of where are all the cancer research funds going? Why has the cure not been found? Why—because it's big business! This beast effects all of us and if you are a man, the odds are closer to 1 in 2 to be newly diagnosed.

Don't be afraid to ask your Oncology team questions. Be your own advocate, no one else cares about your wellbeing as much as you do. So, get your notebook, pen, and your thoughts together and ask away! It's okay to push the envelope and raise the roof. ASK questions, demand answers, and if you're not happy with what you get, then fire the oncologist and find another one. God knows they're out there just waiting for you to walk in their office door.

Make Sure to Note:

• Explore the after-effects of the medications your Oncology Team chooses for you.

• Take off those rose-colored glasses and get ready for some changes

that you may or may not be aware of.

• The following bullet list will help open your eyes and get your

mind-set in the right place.

• Provider visits—How many? Every two weeks or 21 days, or once

a month?

• Lab tests— (blood, urine, and more, which are usually billed

separately);

• Clinic visits for treatments;

• Procedures— (for diagnosis or treatment, which can include room

charges, equipment, different doctors, and more);

• Imaging tests— (such as X-rays, CT scans, and MRI, which may

mean separate bills for radiologist fees, equipment, and any medicines used for the test);

• Radiation treatments— (implants, external radiation, or both);

• Drug costs— (inpatient, outpatient, prescription, non-prescription, and procedure-related);

• Hospital stays— (which can include many types of costs such as

drugs, tests, and procedures, as well as nursing care, doctor visits,

and consults with specialists);

• Surgery— (surgeon, anesthesiologist, pathologist, operating room fees, equipment, medicines, and more);

• Home care— (can include equipment, drugs, visits from specially trained nurses, and more)

Chemotherapy and After Effects

The aftereffects of chemotherapy on the body can be downright harsh. These are commonly referred to as side effects but I can tell you they can be life changing and you may endure them for many years after your treatment is complete.

1. Loss of cognition- referred by chemo patients as chemo brain or chemo fog. Yep, you will forget things! Many patients experience difficulty with memory, basic thought processes, coordination, and mood.

2. Neuropathy in your fingers, hands, and feet. This is no joke. I can't tell you how many glasses I have picked up that mysteriously end up shattered on the floor.

Peripheral neuropathy is tingling in the extremities and maybe accompanied by general fatigue or weakness, shakiness, numbness, or pain. Can also affect basic balance, reflexes, and coordination.

3. Lack of taste, or change of taste, I.E., a metallic taste you can't get rid of and the worst dry mouth ever. In the medical community, this is known as, Xerostomia, which simply means an extremely dry mouth. May cause sores in the soft tissues, difficulty swallowing, and make you more prone to bleeding gums.

4. Nausea—need I say more. Nausea is one of the most common direct effects of chemotherapy, make sure your oncologist gives you several options to help combat this right away.

5. Dehydration—be careful with this one as it can sneak up on you quickly. Make sure to keep water on hand at all times. To help avoid dehydration from vomiting or diarrhea, it's crucial to hydrate as much as possible

6. Fatigue—It's okay to give yourself permission if needed to take much-needed naps. Red blood cells carry the oxygen to your tissues and if your red blood cells aren't getting enough CO_2 then you become tired or fatigued and may have episodes of dizziness, inability to concentrate, feelings of being cold, and overall generalized body weakness.

7. Suppressed Immune system—known as, Neutropenia. Neutropenia is what happens when your body doesn't have enough white blood cells. Lack of these cells increases your risk of infection and reduces the ability to fight cancer.

8. Low platelets—can lead to issues with the blood clotting process. Thrombocytopenia is from a low platelet count. This can cause issues with your menstruation, cause bleeding in your digestive tract that manifests in vomit or stools, and increased incidence of nosebleeds.

9. Diseased Heart—Normal heart size should be about the size of a fist, (I know this first hand). Cardiomyopathy is a weakening of the heart muscle making it harder for your heart to pump blood to the rest of your body.

10. Hair Loss—self-explanatory. Ladies, I will tell you after the initial shock of losing your hair—you can get ready for the day in record time! I learned this a few times on my journey. There are amazing hairpieces and wigs available for both men and woman. Hair loss is known as, Alopecia, and will affect all the hair on your body, (no more shaving)! As a side note—typically your hair will grow back a few weeks after your final chemo infusion Some people experience hair growth during chemo after their initial loss Fingernails and toenails may become weak, split, and become brittle. Discoloration of the nail bed may be a factor as well.

11. Sunburns—may be quicker so make sure to protect your skin by wearing a hat, using an umbrella, and donning sunglasses, whenever possible. Skin Sensitivity or irritation, itchiness, rashes, dryness, and sunburns, are noted in some people. This is the perfect time to obtain a prescription for dark tinted windows in your vehicle to help protect yourself from the sun's rays.

12. Sex Drive-Infertility in both men and women can while undergoing chemotherapy, may also have an impact affecting hormones and sperm count. Women may have a change in menstrual cycles, impact overall sex drive, and cause extreme vaginal dryness, and possible early onset of menopause.

13. Bone Mass density changes—Be cautious of your overall surroundings to reduce the risk of falls. Osteoporosis is the loss of bone mass. Chemotherapy speeds up the process by lowering estrogen levels rapidly resulting in weakening bone marrow.

Four

Sugar, EMF's, Radiation, and Chemotherapy

Truth be known—**CANCER FEEDS ON SUGAR**.
New research shows that sugar doesn't just feed cancer
it causes it!

Sugar does a number of things that are significantly detrimental to the human body. It increases oxidative stress and since cancer is the end result of oxidative stress and inflammation, it needs to be avoided, possibly entirely for some. The huge amounts of sugar the average person consumes on a daily basis is far more than our ancestors would have dreamed of consuming. There should be no surprise that we're seeing higher and higher rates of cancer in the world, and especially in America where consuming vast amounts of sugar is considered normal. Be vigilant in eliminating sugar. It reduces the oxidative stress on the body, and therefore it cuts down inflammation. This improves organ function and deprives cancer of its food source, which limits its ability to grow as an end result.

The first versions of chemotherapy drugs were called, "nitrogen mustards." In 1942, Memorial Sloan-Kettering Cancer Center, secretly began treating breast cancer with this nitrogen mustard. Not one person was ever cured. EMF pollution linked to an increase in cancer. WHAT?

EMF, (Electromagnetic Frequency), pollution has also been consistently linked to cancer increases. The body has its own electromagnetic field and as the body is continually exposed to WIFI, cell phones, dirty AC power, and other sources of electromagnetic radiation, it disrupts the homeostasis of the body's electromagnetic field in negative ways, which can cause a variety of health problems. It's best to avoid electromagnetic radiation whenever possible, through using wired internet connections instead of WiFi, limiting cell phone usage, and using a wired hands-free device to help limit the exposure of the brain to EMF radiation. Being as far away from the wireless "smart meters" as possible, and reducing any dirty power in the house. This can improve sleep, which is necessary for repairing and rejuvenating the body. I'm a huge believer of turning off these devices at night and not having them in our bedrooms.

Did you know that conventional cancer treatments such as chemotherapy and radiation actually promote cancer? Yep, that's right! Something THEY don't want you to be aware of!

Cancer is increasingly becoming a survivable disease; however, treatments cause considerable collateral damage including initiating new, second cancers. What are you kidding me!

My sister and brother Warrior's, let's make sure we do our due diligence and ask questions no matter how or small, silly, or detailed, and let's all empower each other to be informed. Knowledge is power. Did you know the link between chemotherapy, radiation and the development of SECOND cancers has been known for decades? Even the American Cancer Society acknowledges these treatments are carcinogens and that the risk is even higher when both therapies are given together.

Another astonishing fact that your oncologist won't openly share with you is about the chemotherapy drug, 5-fluorouracil, (5-FU), is sometimes referred to by doctors as, "5 feet under," because of its deadly side effects. I ask you how can they knowingly give this to human beings. Would they sit in the recliner and allow this 5-FU to be administered into their port or venerable veins?

In 2004, the Department of Radiation Oncology, Northern Sydney Cancer Centre, Australia, conducted a long-term investigation into the contribution of chemotherapy to 5-year survival in22 major adult malignancies. The results were shocking: The over-all contribution of curative and adjuvant cytotoxic chemotherapy to 5-year survival in adults was estimated to be 2.3% in Australia, and 2.1% in the USA. The study came to the following conclusion: "...It is clear that cytotoxic chemotherapy only makes a minor contribution to cancer survival. To justify the continued funding and availability of drugs used in cytotoxic chemotherapy, a rigorous evaluation of the cost-effectiveness and impact on quality of life is urgently required.

Chemo is massively toxic and kill[s] any rapidly dividing cell, tumor or normal. The three best-selling cancer drugs, worldwide in 2013 were all made by Roche—Rituxan, Herceptin, and Avastin. For all three top chemo drugs sales totaled more than $21 billion. Fred Hutchinson Cancer Research Center, now documents how chemotherapy drugs act as carcinogens. This means they cause cancer which is why, depending on the patient's immune strengthened dosage, within five years, a staggering number die after receiving the chemo treatments that were supposed to have saved them. Let's not forget about Iodine deficiency.

Unfortunately, iodine deficiency in the general population is of pandemic proportions in our modern world due to iodine's displacement in our bodies by environmental toxins such as bromide, pesticides, and food additives. Modern farming techniques have also led to deficiencies of iodine and other minerals in the soil. Crops grown in iodine-deficient soil are deficient in iodine. Now that's not rocket science. Certain diets and lifestyles can also predispose a person to develop iodine deficiency. Those who eat a lot of bakery products such as the breads, pasta, and the list goes on and on, which contain high amounts of bromide, are all at risk. So are vegetarians and those who don't like sea food, vegetables, or salt. It is noted the about 96% of the population is currently iodine deficient. The World Health Organization has recognized iodine deficiency is the world's greatest single cause of preventable mental retardation. Iodine deficiency has been identified as a significant public health problem in129countries and the world's population is affected by an iodine deficiency disorder.

Five

Q & A

Understand that **CANCER is NOT** contagious.

A healthy person cannot "catch" cancer from someone. There is no evidence that close contact or things like sex, kissing, touching, sharing meals, or breathing the same air can spread cancer from one person to another.

Questions and Answers that You May or May not Have Been Aware Of....

Q Why does cancer start in the first place?

A Our bodies are made up of 100 million cells. When every cell is balanced there is no concern, but when the cell structure is interrupted it becomes unbalanced. The result is the cell grows and multiplies quickly. This damaged cell division's end result is a growth commonly known as a tumor. It takes at least 30 cell divisions on one cancer cell to create a tumor that is 1 centimeter in size. This is about half an inch. To be seen on a typical X-ray.

Q Is Cancer inherited?

A Studies have shown that some people are born with a gene mutation that they may have inherited from either their parents. This damaged gene puts that person at a higher risk for developing cancer than most people. This is commonly referred to as hereditary cancer.

Q What percentage of cancer is genetic?

A Studies have shown that inherited gene mutations are thought to play a role in about 5-10% of all cancers see today.

Q Is Cancer a common thing?

A New study show the 1 in 2 people will be diagnosed with some type of cancer by the time they reach the age of 85. Believe it or not, MEN are 1.3 times more likely than women to be diagnosed with cancer.

Q What is the most common type of cancer?

A Breast, Bowel, Lung, Melanoma, Prostate

Q Is it true that cancer spreads after a biopsy?

A Studies of 2000 patients by researchers at the Mayo Clinic's campus in Jacksonville, Florida, have dispelled the myth that biopsies cause cancer to spread. A long-held belief by a number of patients and even some physicians, has been that a biopsy can cause some cancer cells to spread.

*According to research to-date, the following is knowledge-based for the reader to be informed.

Q Can cancer be transmitted sexually?

A Cancer is not contagious, so it won't spread from one person to another. However, some cancers, like cervical, liver, and throat cancer, can be caused by viruses that are spread from one person to another

Q How does cancer spread?

A Some cancerous cells may break away from the tumor and enter the blood stream this allows cancer to spread throughout the body.

Cervical cancer: Virtually all cervical cancers are caused by HPV.

Oropharyngeal cancers: Most oropharyngeal cancers (70%) in

the United States are caused by HPV.

Anal cancer: Over 90% of anal cancers are caused by HPV.

Penile cancer: Most penile cancers (over 60%) are caused by HPV.

Vaginal cancer: Most vaginal cancers (75%) are caused by HPV.

Vulvar cancer: Most vulvar cancers (70%) are caused by HPV.

In the United States, high-risk HPVs cause 3% of all cancers in women and 2% of all cancers in men, resulting in about 43,000 HPV-related cancers each year.

Q Can a woman spread cervical cancer to a man?

A HPV/Genital Warts—HPV Infection in men. Much of the information about HPV virus, centers on women, since having the virus increases their risk of getting cervical cancer, However, male HPV virus can cause health problems.

Q Can you get cancer from sperm?

A Men undergoing any chemotherapy treatments should avoid

impregnating their partner and for some time after treatment concludes due to the fact that the chemotherapy agent may cause unknown damage in the DNA in sperm cells. Please take note again that your cancer treatment does not make sex dangerous. You should inquire with your oncologist for further information.

Q How long is chemo in sperm?

A In most cases, chemotherapy is excreted in the body fluids for up to 48 hours after treatment, However, some agents can be found in excrement for up to seven days.

Q What are the warning signs I should be aware of with cancer?

A The following symptoms may be associated with the likelihood

of a Cancer diagnosis:

· A sore that doesn't heal.

· Bladder and Bowel changes.

· Cough that won't go away

· Difficultly Swallowing

· Hoarseness

· Indigestion

· Lump in the breast or another part of the body

· Obvious changes noted in a wart or mole

· Unusual bleeding or discharge

Q Can exercise cause my cancer to spread?

A Increased blood flow from exercise has been found to reduce cancer to grow and spread. Cancer warriors are often advised to exercise. Consult your Oncology team should you have questions.

Q Is it possible to cure cancer completely?

A If the cancer is gone after treatment and there is no longer evidence of it then this is referred to as a complete remission. Don't confuse this with a cure, because of the chance that there may still be some cancer cells in the body, blood, etc., that the oncologist is unable to see. A partial remission means that cancer has shrunk from its original finding.

Q What if I refuse the treatment offered for my particular cancer?

A Should this be your choice, you would be offered Supportive Care or Palliative Care which is care offered to help keep patients with cancer from having to deal with uncomfortable pain, nausea, or other symptoms. Also, be aware of the Hospice Care option as well.

Q Did you know that you have the right to obtain ALL your medical records?

A As a patient, you have the legal right to inspect, review, and receive a copy of your medical records from your providers.

Q What is neuropathy?

A Neuropathy is a side effect from some of the chemotherapy treatments if effects hand, feet and can be painful at times. I've heard that soaking your hands in ice water will help.

Q Does CBD help with the pain?

A CBD has proven to be effective for the nerve pain that you may experience. CBD and high potency THC oil together is known to kill cancer cells. CBD used alone is known to help control pain issues. CBD oil is sublingual.

Q What is the muscle cramping all about?

A There could be a magnesium deficiency. You could try eating raw pumpkin seeds to help keep your magnesium levels up. Topical magnesium spray is available also and works immediately.

Q Can I look into alternative therapies and what is available?

A Of course, you can! This is your journey and you are the driver. Explore the following: High dose Vitamin C IV infusions, Vitamin K3, and B17. Apparently, some of these modalities are not legal in the USA but in Mexico, they are having great success with their treatment protocols. Also, look into use of turmeric and cat's claw herb. Carnivora is another good herb. This is what President Reagan took when he had cancer while in office. You can look into the benefits of using Colloidal Silver.

Q Does an alkaline diet help?

A An Alkaline diet will aid in killing cancer and help to keep it from coming back. Drinking alkaline water is beneficial as well.

Q What is Ozone therapy?

A Cancer cells die when exposed to oxygen, (cancer cells are an aerobic). There are many oxygen and ozone treatments, however, this article will discuss two of the best known and most effective "Stage IV" treatments—infusion bottle and ozone I.V. Ozone therapy using an infusion bottle, involves removing part of the blood from the body, saturating this blood with oxygen(I.E. ozone—O3), then putting this oxygen-rich blood back into the body. An ozone I.V. simply injects a fluid saturated with ozone into the blood. Both treatments work by getting oxygen into the body. The Ozone RHP technique, puts ozone gas directly into the bloodstream.

Q What is hyperthermia?

A Hyperthermia, (also called thermal therapy or thermotherapy), is a type of cancer treatment in which body tissue is exposed to high temperatures, (up to 113°F). Research has shown that high temperatures can damage and kill cancer cells, usually with minimal injury to normal tissues.

Q Is B17 really effective?

A Yes, it is. Feel free to do your research on this one.

Q What will help with the metallic taste in my mouth?

A Try switching from metal silverware to plastic.

Q What is Dendritic Cell Therapy?

A This is the process of using our own cells and essentially creating a Vaccine

Q What is the RGCC test, (Greece test)

A This is a test that sends your blood to Greece to be tested to see what would be effective in your particular cancer case.

As a side note, this is usually ordered from a Natural path doctor or a Natural path Oncologist.

Q Does lemongrass tea help with nausea?

A Yes, it has proven to be quite effective in knocking out nausea feeling from chemotherapy and radiation treatments.

Q How do I pay for chemotherapy treatment?

A According to the American Cancer Society, Medicare Part B and most insurance companies reimburse at least a part of cost associated with chemotherapy.

Six

Doctor Lingo

This is deep and contains important information so listen up...

Cancer staging is a key marker to determine the extent of the disease from which a treatment strategy will be implemented. Ranging from stage 0 to stage 4, these stages assess the size of the tumor, lymph node involvement, and whether cancer has spread. The stage is determined after the tumor and or lymph nodes are removed and examined by a pathologist.

Most cancers that involve a tumor are staged in five broad groups. Other kinds of cancer, for example—blood cancers, lymphoma, and brain cancer have their own staging systems. But they all tell you how advanced the cancer is.

Stage 0

Means there is NO cancer, only abnormal cells with the potential to become cancer. This is also referred to as a Carcinoma in Situ.

Stage I

Means the cancer is small and only located in ONE area. This is also commonly referred to and called early-stage cancer.

Stage II and III

Mean the cancer is larger and HAS GROWN into nearby tissues or lymph nodes.

Stage IV

Means cancer HAS SPREAD to other parts of your body. This is referred as advanced cancer or metastatic cancer.

Tumor, node, and metastasis is-TNM System:

Another factor your doctor probably will use to determine your overall cancer stage is the TNM system. Your oncologist will measure each of these and give it a number or an "X" if a measurement can't be determined. The symbols are a bit different for each type of cancer, but this is generally what they mean overall:

Tumor (T)

"T" followed by a number from 0-4, tells how LARGE the tumor is and sometimes where it's located. T0 means there is NO MEASURABLE tumor. The higher the number, the bigger the tumor.

Node (N)

"N" followed by a number from 0-3, tells if cancer has spread to your lymph nodes. These are glands that filter things like viruses and bacteria before they can infect other parts of your body. N0 means lymph nodes aren't involved. A higher number means the cancer is in more lymph nodes, farther away from the original tumor.

Metastasis (M)

"M" is followed by either 0 or 1. It indicates if cancer has spread to organs and tissues in other parts of your body. A0 means it hasn't,

and a 1 means it has.

More Important Information:

Grade

This is how cancer cells look under a microscope. Low grade

means they look a lot like normal cells. High grade means they look

very abnormal. Low-grade cancer cells grow more slowly and are

less likely to spread than high-grade.

Location

Where the tumor is in your body may make it harder to treat.

Tumor markers

These are things in your blood or urine that are at higher levels

when you have certain kinds of cancer.

Genetics

The DNA of the cancer cells can tell your doctor if it's likely to spread and what treatment may work. Once your Oncologist has all this information and has assigned numbers to T, N, and M, they can determine your overall stage. A side note: your cancer stage will typically stay the same as when you were first diagnosed. For example, if you're diagnosed with stage II lung cancer, that's what it will be called, whether it spreads or goes into remission. That's when cancer cells are gone. In a few cases, your oncologist may run a battery of tests and may re-stage your cancer if they find a reason to do so.

Understanding the difference between how growth differs in benign and malignant tumors. Benign tumors develop from healthy cells and they usually grow slowly—over months, perhaps even years. Benign tumors NEVER infiltrate neighboring tissues. Benign tumors can occasionally reach impressive sizes, pushing or squeezing other organs, but they never spread into those organs. These tumors can be painful, uncomfortable, can be seen with the naked eye, and can often be felt or even cause a cosmetic defect. Benign tumors can also cause significant health problems, especially if they develop in, for example, the brain. Benign tumors are usually contained within a fibrous capsule, so they have clear borders that are tangible, (smooth contoured formations that are clearly separate from surrounding tissues), or visible in an ultrasound, X-ray examination, CT scan, or an MRI. Benign tumors occasionally secrete hormones or other biologically active substances, which can affect various functions of the body. Benign tumors never metastasize in lymph nodes or in other distant tissues or organs. For this reason, they are not fatal, but due to their location or size, can cause significant complaints and symptoms. After they've been surgically removed, they usually don't return, unless, in rare cases, the tumor wasn't completely removed. This may happen even though a surgeon may cut outside the borders it would take just one cell to escape and cause havoc in our system.

The hard TRUTH regarding malignant tumors

Malignant tumors develop from cancer cells and they usually grow faster. However, there are certain tumors that grow slowly and it's even possible that a person can die from a completely different cause with a tumor firmly lodged inside them. This can happen with tumors of the prostate and many other cancerous pathogens, (non-invasive formations that don't grow in neighboring tissue and have pronounced cellular atypia, or similarity to a malignant tumor). However, it would be wrong to put one's faith in this possibility, because we can never know the exact moment when this situation can change. Malignant tumors grow directly into neighboring tissues, literally drilling through them destroying natural borders and spreading via the path of least resistance. In addition, malignant tumors have a unique characteristic their cells can separate themselves from their respective groups and spread throughout the lymphatic or circulatory systems, as well as simply peeling away and spreading to various natural cavities. In this way, for example, tumors often grow through the walls of the stomach or intestines where they can float freely in the abdominal cavity. After surgery, there's always a risk that the tumor can return over time. Then we're talking about relapse or a metastasis.

Even after destroying 99.99% of all cancer cells, over time the remaining 0.01% is enough to begin, under the right circumstances multiplying and spreading once again.

Volume Doubling

The following information is just for your knowledge it is not meant to cause you any anxiety in any way, I simply added it for people who are curious about Volume doubling and what it exactly means.

Volume doubling is the time it takes for the mass of the tumor to double in size. However, this time can vary between different types of tumors. Calculations derived from retrospective studies of patients with lung cancer tumors revealed that the volume doubling time was on average 223 days for fast-growing tumors and 545 for slow-growing tumors. Furthermore, the average number of days was 303 for adenocarcinomas, 77 for squamous cell carcinomas, and only 70 for small cell lung cancer.

The prognosis was better for those patients whose volume doubling times were over 200 days. It's been estimated that for a tumor to grow to a mass of 1 cm3, an average of 30 volume doubling times are necessary or 30 full growth periods between two successful mitoses, (the process of cell division). So, if the volume doubling time is around 75 days, then 30 doubling times will take longer than 6 years. That means that even fast-growing tumors REQUIRE several years to reach sizes that can be detected by medical diagnostic imaging methods.

FACT:

It's been determined that the average volume doubling time for acute leukemia is roughly 2 weeks, 3 months for breast cancer and 6–12 months for myeloma. By comparison, the average doubling time for the normal mucous membrane cells of the rectum is 24 hours. It has also been determined that after 39–42 episodes of doubling, the size of the tumor is so large that it is lethal to the patient. Scary to think about however, important to give a minute of thought. The mass of tumor cells depends on the balance between the formation of new cells and the loss of existing cells, (surgery, radiation, drug therapy).

We can hope that therapy will significantly reduce the number of detectable tumor cells, but even if only a small amount of cells remain intact and they become active overtime, the cancer can begin to spread once again and this time we won't know its volume doubling time or how quickly the disease will advance. This is one reason why scientists have such high hopes for immunotherapy— to awaken and stimulate dormant immunity, so it can take appropriate action when a new clone army of cancer cells is born inside the body. So, here's something to ponder about—if the tumor has already been in the host body for at least 5–10 years then how is it possible to have an early diagnosis of the cancer. I believe this to be a bit misleading.

This is also the reason why it's not always possible to successfully treat all early-stage cancers and to reduce their mortality rate. Biologically speaking, the term early essentially means late. This is why not all small tumors are considered to be early-stage cancers, especially since they have lived half of their biological lives inside a person's body. This is also the reason why mammogram screenings haven't reduced mortality rates as much as was originally hoped. However, they can significantly reduce the spread of the tumor and prolong life. Screening results for cervical and intestinal cancers are different, as they often search for precancerous pathogens, (conditions such as cervical dysplasia, colon polyps, or adenomas, which, if left untreated, can lead to cancer). By surgically removing or treating them in some other manner, the patient is spared from their potential transformation into cancerous tumors. Mammograms, on the other hand, essentially attempt to detect what we can call small cancers, because we still haven't identified this organ's precancerous conditions. With today's available detection methods, not all tumors that have been identified in their early stages can have a positive prognosis, because it's possible that dissemination, or the spread of the tumor cells throughout the body, has already occurred.

The introduction of routine PET/CT, (positron emission tomography), scans in oncology only proves this assertion as patients with tumors that were supposedly caught in their early stages have, unfortunately, already spread to other parts of the body, requiring a change in their treatment plans. If it was possible to detect tumors when they are only 2 mm2, (roughly 107 cells), instead of at the current size of1 cm2 (roughly 109 cells), this would extend the patient's monitoring period by about three years. These people would then be able to live for an extra three years as cancer patients, instead of just average citizens. In medical statistics this period is called the Leadtime bias. We know that tumors metastasize at roughly the same pace as the initial tumor. So, for example, if the primary tumor's growth to a detectable size, (1 cm3), occurred over the course of 10 years, then roughly the same period of time will be necessary until its metastasis is determined and, likewise, if the primary tumor developed over the course of three years, then we can expect the metastasis to develop over the next three years after the diagnosis. Does that make sense? Therefore, so-called late metastases, aren't actually late, but rather metastases that have grown in accordance with the original tumor's pace of growth. From a biological standpoint, the generally accepted five-year life expectancy for many slow-growing tumors, (breast, prostate, kidney, intestinal, etc.), is false.

The volume doubling time is a much more precise measurement

for tumors. The life expectancy for an untreated patient with a tumor whose volume doubling time is 10 days can live for another 100 days,(a little longer than 3 months), but if the volume doubling time is 200 days, then we can expect the patient to live at least another 2,000 days or roughly 6 years. Tumors with very fast volume doubling times include testicular tumors. Unfortunately, the process occurs quite quickly, which is why it's important to begin aggressive therapy as quickly as possible to reduce the mass of the cancer cells. With that being said we need to get right in our spiritual beliefs and there's no time like the present. Okay enough with the hard facts let's move on. It is okay to cry, get mad, stomp your feet, pound on the wall, or curse if it will make you feel better! Give yourself permission to be mad at the world and then pick yourself up and get it together. You need to be STRONG in your battle to become a Warrior Survivor.

Seven

The First Oncologist Appointment

An Interview with an Oncologist

That's right—remember you are interviewing your doctor. You need to feel confident that they know what they are doing. After all, it is called practicing medicine! Just because they have the white coat on, perfect hair, and a folder and pen in their hand doesn't necessarily mean they are a good doctor, let alone have a good bedside manner. Should you not jive with this particular individual, don't give it a second thought to interview another. Remember physicians can fire us as a patient and we have the power to fire them and seek treatment somewhere else. Okay, just so you know your first cancer appointment can be a bit overwhelming. Your head may be spinning in so many directions it doesn't know which way is up and you may be filled with a host of fears, worries, and questions. I've created this checklist as a starting reference point for you to take with you to your first appointment. Read through it and get your wheels upstairs moving, that way when you walk out of the oncology office you walk with the Confidence, Empowerment, and Knowledge, to get you through your Battle with the Beast you are about to endure.

Get prepared for your appointment

Sit down take as much time as you need and write down everything that is running around in your mind at that very moment. This will prove helpful with getting your questions and concerns in order to help give you a point of reference to start from. When you call the office for your appointment, inquire if there is a nurse navigator to help assist you with the process of being new to the office. Nurse navigators assist with setting patients, I refer to us as clients into support groups of all kinds, meals on wheels, cancer connection Facebook groups, these folks are an invaluable to us as a resource. Ask someone that you trust if it's your wish that they accompany you to your appointment. If anything, they can be your secretary and write the answers to all of your questions—but of course make sure you can read their writing. Again, don't be afraid to talk. In fact, talk a lot! Ask anything that pops into your mind after all it's YOUR life we are talking about here. It's okay to talk candid and to be frank with your oncologist and the cancer care team, and it helps if you know what to ask.

Your questions may look like this:

- How much experience do you have with treating my type of cancer?
- How many people with my type of cancer have you treated within the past year?
- What hospitals do you work with?
- Are you board certified? In what specialty or sub-specialty?
- Do you work closely with other specialists and health care providers who could be part of my cancer treatment team?
- What kind of cancer do I have?
- Is the kind of cancer I have treatable?
- What stage is my cancer?
- Where is my cancer located?
- Has my cancer spread?
- Is this cancer considered terminal?
- Is my cancer a common type or is it rare in nature?
- What are my treatment options?
- Is my cancer considered to be a rare or common type?
- What stage is it?

- What exactly does that mean to me as a patient and you as my Oncologist?
- Can my cancer be cured?
- What is the standard protocol for the type of cancer I have and
- What are the downsides?
- What are the goals for my treatment plan?
- Will I be in pain and if so, what medications are available to ease my discomfort?
- If not is there possibility to it be controlled?
- When should I tell my family?
- Will I need to have any further testing at this time and if so what exactly?
- What are my treatment options?
- What are your recommendations and why do you believe they will work for me?
- Can you recommend a colleague for a second opinion or a third?
- Where do I receive my actual treatments?
- How do I pay for all of this?
- Does my insurance cover any or part of it or do I have to exhaust?
- my savings, 401k, etc.?
- Do they schedule close to my home or will I be driving a few? hours for it?
- May I have a tour of the facility before starting my treatment
- program?
- Do you know if this is a genetic link to this type of cancer?
- Do you recommend diagnostic testing for my family?
- What side effects should I be made of aware of before, during, and after, my treatments?
- How will cancer treatment affect my daily life?
- What do you suggest to keep me in the best version of myself? during all of this?
- Should I continue using supplements, vitamins, minerals

etc?

- And if not why? Listen to their opinion and then go do your own research on this. Be informed.
- What does this diagnosis mean exactly?
- What about any new clinical trials? Would I be such a candidate?
- What support groups do you recommend, if any?
- What are my next steps?

Cancer treatment isn't easy, it's a bit overwhelming for the strongest of us!

Eight

Michelle's Tips to keeping things organized...

For some of us, we may be super organized in our careers, but at home you can't remember where you put something even though when you initially put it there, you swore you would!

Start a file where you can keep copies of all test results, medication, nutrition, and therapy tips, and any other information that relates to your type of cancer, treatment, or healthcare team. Keep a running list of any questions that occur to you as you move forward, or side effects or problems that develop so you can discuss them with your Oncology care team. Talk with your family about what is happening, perhaps even bringing certain members to appointments so they have a better understanding of your disease and how it can affect you physically and psychologically.

Your treatment plan will be constructed based upon this

information that will come from the pathology report. Your oncologist will oversee all aspects of your treatment including surgery, chemotherapy, medication, radiation, and recovery. Many people take vitamins and mineral supplements to support optimal health and nutrition, but first and foremost, I do believe we should all strive to consume high-quality food. Some high-dose antioxidant supplements can lessen the effectiveness of cancer treatment, so it is important to discuss any vitamin supplement usage with your oncologist or your dietitian. Again, be informed. Many patients with cancer are already in pain from the disease.

Cancer treatment and/or surgery can lessen or even alleviate this pain. When needed, there are pain management physicians who specialize in helping to minimize pain for patients with cancer and who are undergoing therapy. The only person who should make the decision to share their battle of a lifetime is the patient. Ask your oncologist if he or she would mind be part of the conversation with the family in order to help address questions and concerns. If you choose not to take anyone, simply ask if you can record the conversation. Most of us have some kind of smart phone device that we can do this with a push of a button, and if you've never done it before Google it. Those who are more private and/or wish to maintain as normal life as possible throughout this process, choose not to share their diagnosis. There is no right or wrong way to do this. I believe it's whatever you can handle at the moment. Don't allow the pressure of others judging you during this time. Remember, others' opinions about you, is none of your business. So, carry on! Once you understand the kind of cancer you are dealing with you can better understand your oncologist recommendation for the plan to treat it. Of course, your age, general health, the location of cancer, and other contributing factors, will all be considered for your particular treatment plan.

Please be aware that not all cancers are the same and some of us may have to make choices for our particular cancer treatment plan to have the best possible outcome. Some treatment plans are more aggressive than others. Make sure to inquire regarding the downside or side effects to ensure you are fully informed. Patient and family member support is vital to assisting with the physical, emotional, and financial challenges, that lie ahead. Every family needs to take advantage of these services, including palliative care, which helps to lighten the responsibilities and lessen stress for everyone involved.

Michelle's tips to help get you through the day.

Here's a quick list of things to stock up on before your chemo infusions begin:

• Dissolving Nausea Medicine

• Gummy Vitamins

• Starburst Peppermint candies

• Peppermint Essential Oil

• Eucalyptus shampoo

• Loofah washcloth

• Unscented baby wipes

• Milk of Magnesia- cherry/mint flavor)

• Hand & Foot cream—your hands and feet will crack—no doubt about it

• Mineral oil

• MiraLAX for constipation issue

• Aquaphor -feet, scars

• Ginger Snaps- helps combat digestive distress, churning, nausea

• Aloe- scalp and body—helps to cool and feel a little better as your skin may become dry

• Cooling Sunblock

• Fleet mineral oil enema—for constipation

• Caregivers or loved ones that know what DEHYDRATION looks like. This can be dangerous.

• IV fluids with potassium, magnesium, steroids, & anti-nausea meds

• Ensure nutritional drinks

• Premier Protein Drinks

• Vitamin Water

• Popsicle's

• Anything to help keep you hydrated.

Extra tidbits of info

• Combat neuropathy with lotion.

• For neuropathy, soak your hands in ice water

• I wish I'd have known to put lotion on my hands and feet every day. By the time I figured it out, my hands and feet were cracked and bleeding. My skin and calluses were sloughing off. It took some industrial strength Eucerin Healing Repair cream to help elevate this problem. I looked like a lizard!

• Watch your grip on hand railings. If you get, neuropathy, numbness in the hands and feet can be tricky to navigate.

• You may go through some serious emotional episodes.

• Diarrhea may follow constipation so if you wish to keep some baby wipes on hand.

• Ask your doctor for a prescription for the Miracle Mouth wash as you may develop sores in your mouth.

• Vomiting to hard may cause vocal cord damage.

• Your vision may change.

• Steroids during chemo make you gain weight, (may be good for some, but for me not so much).

• Get your teeth checked.

• Your gums may bleed.

• If your scalp starts tingling, you may be getting ready to lose your hair, and remember it's okay, honestly, on the bright side of things, this makes getting ready much faster, plus it usually will grow back sometimes in a different color or texture.

• Get head wraps as your head will get cold believe it or not.

• Wear sunscreen on your head.

• Your taste buds may change and things may have a metallic taste.

• Chemo brain is a real thing.

• You will be tired so sleep often.

• After your treatment, rest, and stay hydrated.

• It's okay to say, No. Take care of yourself.

• You may lose your hair remember—it's okay it WILL grow back!

My daughter once told me, "It's okay mom, hair is like grass. It will grow back—just give it some water. "Listen for just a second, okay, they've given you the news, went over your treatment options, discussed your date of attack to begin, and you're stuck not knowing for sure what to do. STOP, BREATHE AND TAKE 5. It's okay to be overwhelmed with emotions, and if you weren't feeling a little uneasy, I'd wonder what was wrong with you— besides the obvious. Give yourself permission to consider all your treatment options and then after your decision is made, relax, it's going to be a bumpy ride, but it will all be okay! I promise. I hate to break this to you, but hey, it's the cold-hearted truth, the side effects of chemotherapy will differ from person to person. Some will have severe side effects and then there's the lucky one who don't notice too many changes. For the rest of you on this side of the spectrum, I'll enlighten you with known side effects reported by other warriors like yourself. My question that I pose to you, ask your oncologist to go over this list, and then ask if they would walk your path and then pay special attention to their answer. Next, ask them why they don't arm us with a list of all the possible side effects from our chemotherapy and radiation on our initial consultation. Would it be that it would pose too many questions and they simply don't have enough time carved out to answer? Or could it be that they are afraid we'd run out the office never to return!

Possible side effects

- Anemia
- Appetite Loss
- Attention, Thinking, or Memory Problems
- Bleeding Problems
- Blocked Intestine or Gastrointestinal Obstruction
- Clotting Problems
- Constipation
- Diarrhea
- Difficulty Chewing
- Difficulty Swallowing or Dysphagia
- Dry Mouth or Xerostomia
- Edema or Fluid Retention

- Fatigue

- Fluid Around the Lungs or Malignant Pleural Effusion

- Fluid in the Abdomen or Ascites

- Fluid in the Arms or Legs, or Lymphedema

- Hair Loss or Alopecia

- Hand-Foot Syndrome or Palmar-Plantar Erythrodysesthesia

- Headaches

- Hormone Deprivation Symptoms: Men

- Hypercalcemia

- Infection

- Menopausal Symptoms: Women

- Mental Confusion or Delirium

- Mouth Sores or Mucositis

- Nausea and Vomiting

- Nervous System Side Effects

- Neutropenia

- Osteoporosis

- Pain

- Sexual Problems

- Skin Conditions

- Shortness of Breath or Dyspnea

- Skin Reactions to Targeted Therapies

• Sleeping Problems: Hypersomnia or Somnolence Syndrome
or Nightmares

• Sleeping Problems: Insomnia

• Superior Vena Cava Syndrome

• Taste Changes

• Thrombocytopenia

• Urinary Incontinence

• Weight Gain

• Weight Loss

A little something extra to think about

Did you know that the success rates for cancer range from

3%–90% for the same type of cancer? Most people go with
conven-

tional treatment, (the 3% treatments), because they do not know

about alternative treatments which have up to a 90% success rate.

Most doctors that were taught western medicine continue to

only think one way. They are conditioned that the old black and

white books are the word and they must follow nothing else. They

are not inclined to think outside the box, or color outside the
lines—

even a little bit. Honestly, what would this hurt? I pose this
question,

if it was your loved one with a diagnosis of cancer or better yet, you

as the doctor, was diagnosed, would you be inclined to step outside

the box and explore other avenues of cancer-killing treatment?

Did you know that the average overall contribution chemotherapy gives you is only a 3% survival rate for some cancers?

That is ludicrous! If cancer patients were made aware of that

upfront do you honestly think that you would choose that option

for your treatment plan? Most people would be better off doing

nothing at all to treat their cancer than to submit their bodies to

this toxic treatment and all the side effects that go along with it.

This statistic makes my heart ache, but the proof is in the pudding.

Do your research and look up Australian and American traditional

medicine, "5-year survival", charts and see what the 5-year cure rate

is for your type of cancer.

(Cure rate is defined by surviving 5 years after diagnosis)

Clinical Oncology (2004, p.549–560):

Oncology Cure Rates

Another fact worth sharing

The most common cancers linked to chemotherapy drugs are AML, (acute myelogenous leukemia), and MDS, (myelodysplastic syndrome). The news of ABC's Good Morning America host Robin

Robert's diagnosis of MDS is a perfect example.

Radiation therapy has been linked to the occurrence of solid tumors of the lung, stomach, and bone, and to various types of leukemia such as AML (acute myelogenous leukemia), CML (chronic myelogenous leukemia), and ALL, (acute lymphoblastic leukemia).

Sadly, many oncologists do not inform their patients that the treatments they prescribe could possibly lead to a second cancer. Yes, you heard me right.

Chemotherapy and Second Cancers

Chemotherapy targets the DNA of cancer cells, specifically rapidly dividing cells. However, in the process it also impacts healthy cells. The risk is dose and treatment-duration related.

How Long Has It Been Known That Chemotherapy an d Radiation Can Lead to Second Cancers?

The link between chemotherapy and radiation and the development of second cancers has been known for decades! Even the American Cancer Society acknowledges that chemotherapy and radiotherapy are carcinogens and may increase risk for developing a second cancer, and that the risk is even higher when both therapies are given together. Yet still this information is not typically shared with patients or is severely downplayed by oncologists – unless you ask specific pointed questions about your proposed radiation therapy and/or chemo.

Second cancers are cancers unrelated to the original cancer, which can be triggered by the very same imbalances or cancer-causing agents that led to the first cancer. In fact, doctors sometimes refer to the risk of a second cancer as "friendly fire"—that is treatment for one cancer resulting in the initiation of a second cancer.

How in God's name could any doctor fail to mention to a patient the possibility that second cancers can be created by the very cancer treatment they are administering?

We live in a Toxic Environment are you glowing yet?!

We must be informed about our exposure to toxins.

This includes ALL fast foods, the vast majority of prepackaged foods, (check the ingredients), and foods that contain anti-nutrients, (the biggest offenders being wheat especially, but all grains in general, dairy, except butter and ghee, soy, legumes, and nightshades). Fast foods are loaded with agricultural toxins, (primarily produced by Monsanto), and heavy metals, so this introduces a significant toxic burden on the body.

Fast foods are inflammatory and lack nutrition, so in addition to putting stress on the body they don't provide the nutrition that the body needs to be able to heal. As well, reducing the toxins within your immediate environment, (household cleaners, personal care products, soaps, shampoos, perfumes, non-stick cooking pans, etc.), and anything you use in your house, car, office, and especially put on your skin, will also help reduce the toxic burden on your body. Detoxing and improving organ function, (especially the liver and kidneys), will likely be essential as part of healing from cancer.

Next, related to toxic situations, toxic people, and toxic emotions, are environmental toxins. Due to industrialization and numerous mega corporations with a psychopathic mentality and no concern for polluting the planet, the world has become quite significantly toxic. There are a wide array of environmental toxins, ranging from synthetic chemicals, artificial sweeteners, flavors, and fats, radioactive elements, (from nuclear waste and nuclear explosions), heavy metals, natural toxins that are released from energy and manufacturing industries, along with natural toxins due to parasitic microorganisms that are in our bodies, and even our own waste from metabolic processes in the body.

These toxins put a stress load on the body and cause organ dysfunction and even damage, so reducing and eliminating the introduction of toxins into the body is a key to healing the body. Now that you've been empowered with information Go Fight that

Battle and WIN! Life is precious. Live it to the fullest. Go make those memories. Rejoice in the good days and celebrate the rough ones as they are just a reminder that we are

still CHOSEN to live this life!

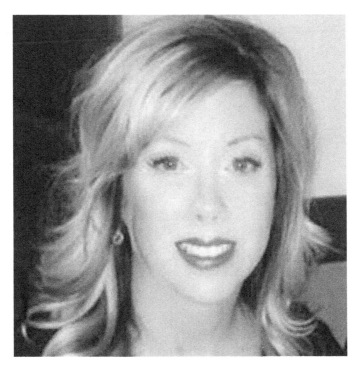

Michelle is a three-time cancer survivor and continues to push the envelope of her Oncology Team! She is truly a one-of-a-kind patient. She writes from confidence and first-hand experience about going in with your questions ready and loaded to interview the doctor. After all, you as the patient, are employing them so you both should be on the same team with winning goal and end result in mind. If not, continue to interview, and if needed fire the doctor and move to a professional that has your best interest at heart.

This book is to Inspire, Empower and Educate you!

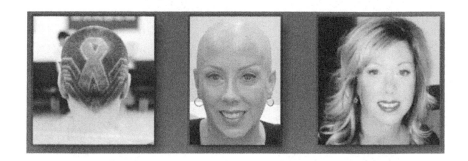

"The Chosen Warrior"

Made in United States
Orlando, FL
22 May 2023